Succeeding Saffi

Using switch scanning to find the right one

Created by Luke Thompson

Co-author Caroline Bennett

Illustrated by Kat Willott

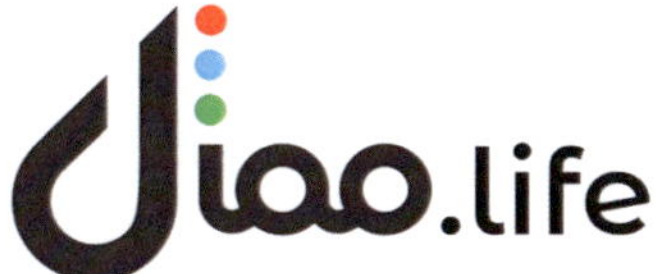

Scan the QR codes to access the digital book or listen to the audio book.

The Seven Stages of Switch Development

Succeeding Saffi is part of the Switch Heroes, social stories created to support switch-users with their Switch progression. The Switch Heroes series is part of the Seven Stages of Switch Development, created by Occupational Therapist and AT specialist Luke Thompson.

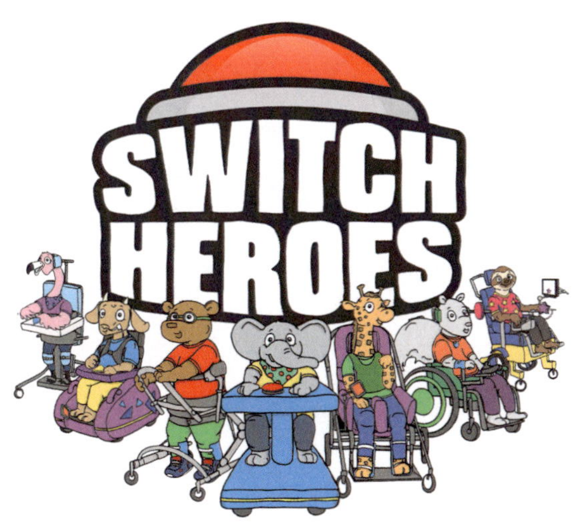

Her switch is pink and oval

Have a look and see

Of course, it's Saffi Squirrel

Who else would it be?

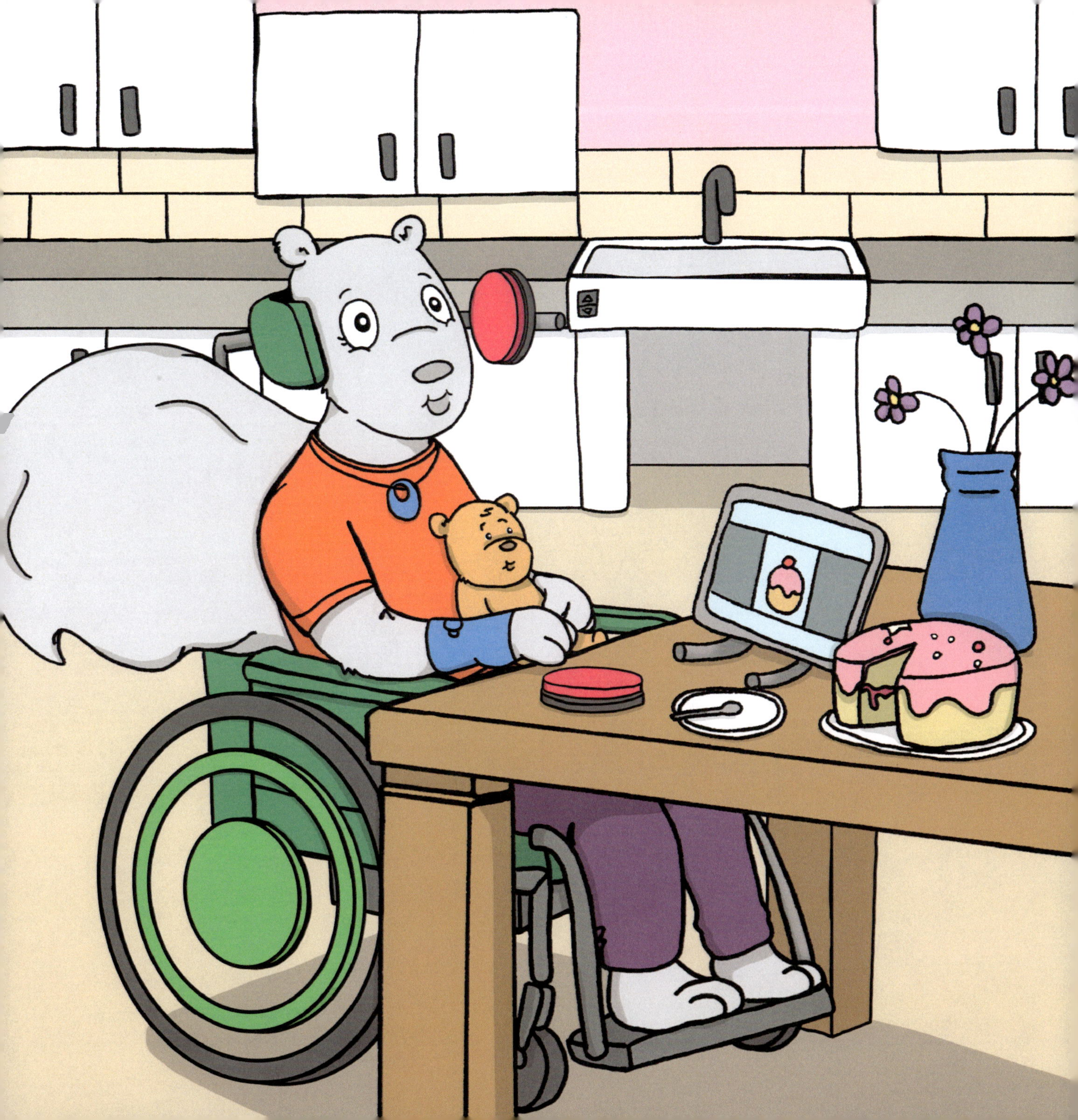

Her switches are in place

Where they need to be

One on her headrest,
one on the table

Have a look and see

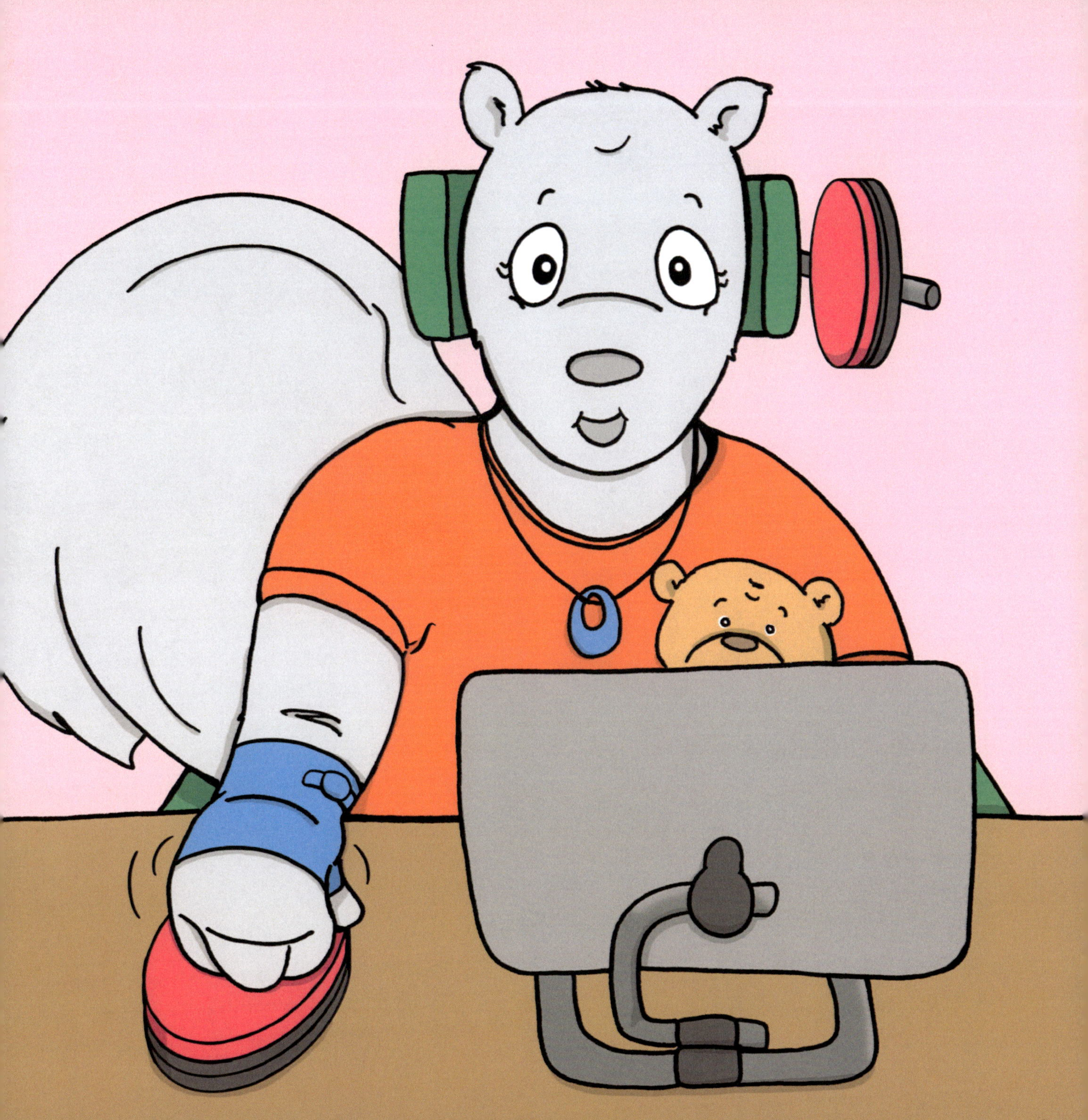

When she's asked the question

"What shall we feed teddy?"

Saffi uses switches

To get her answer ready

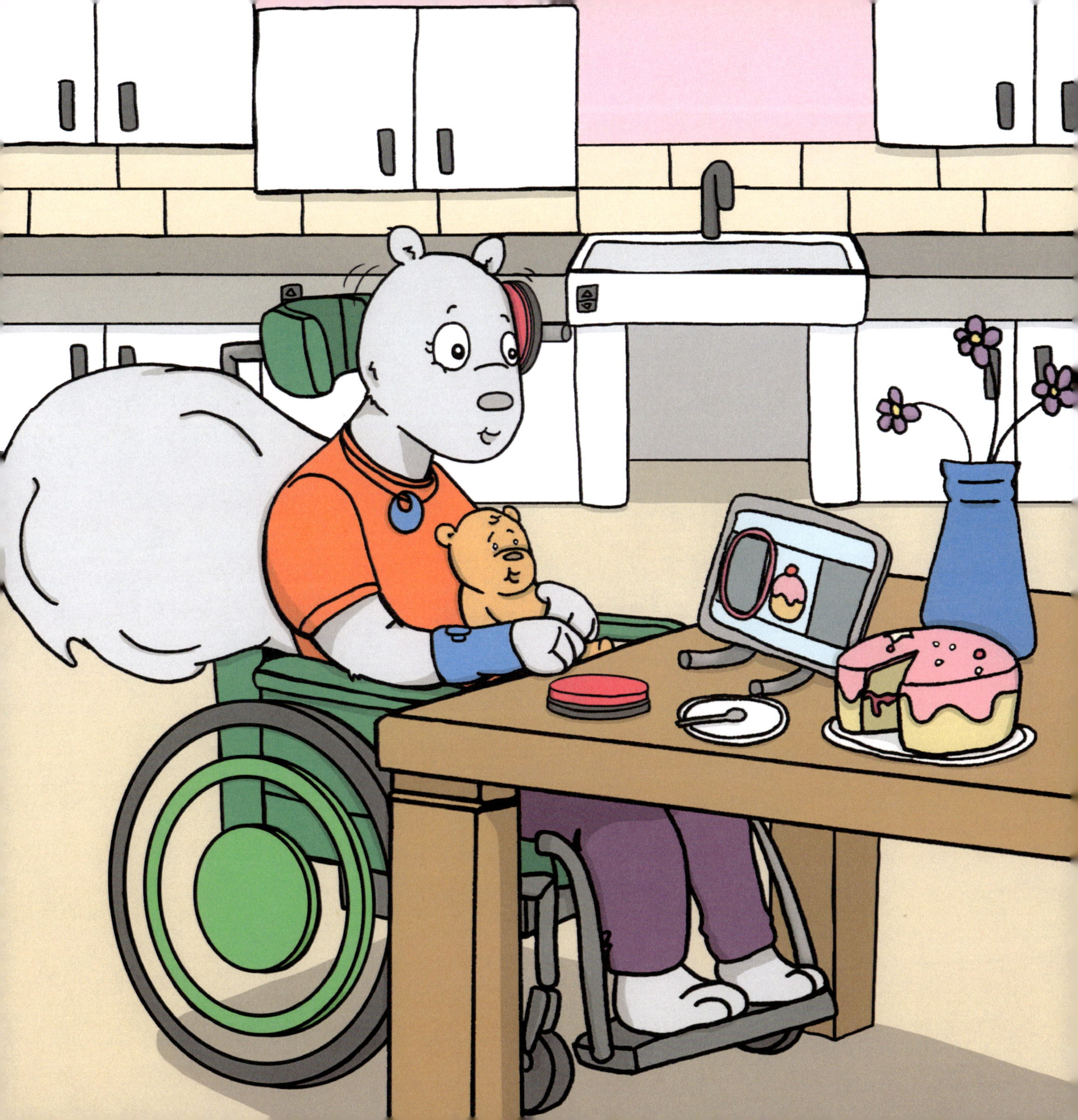

She uses switches carefully

To scan and make a choice

She selects option three

But her device plays no voice

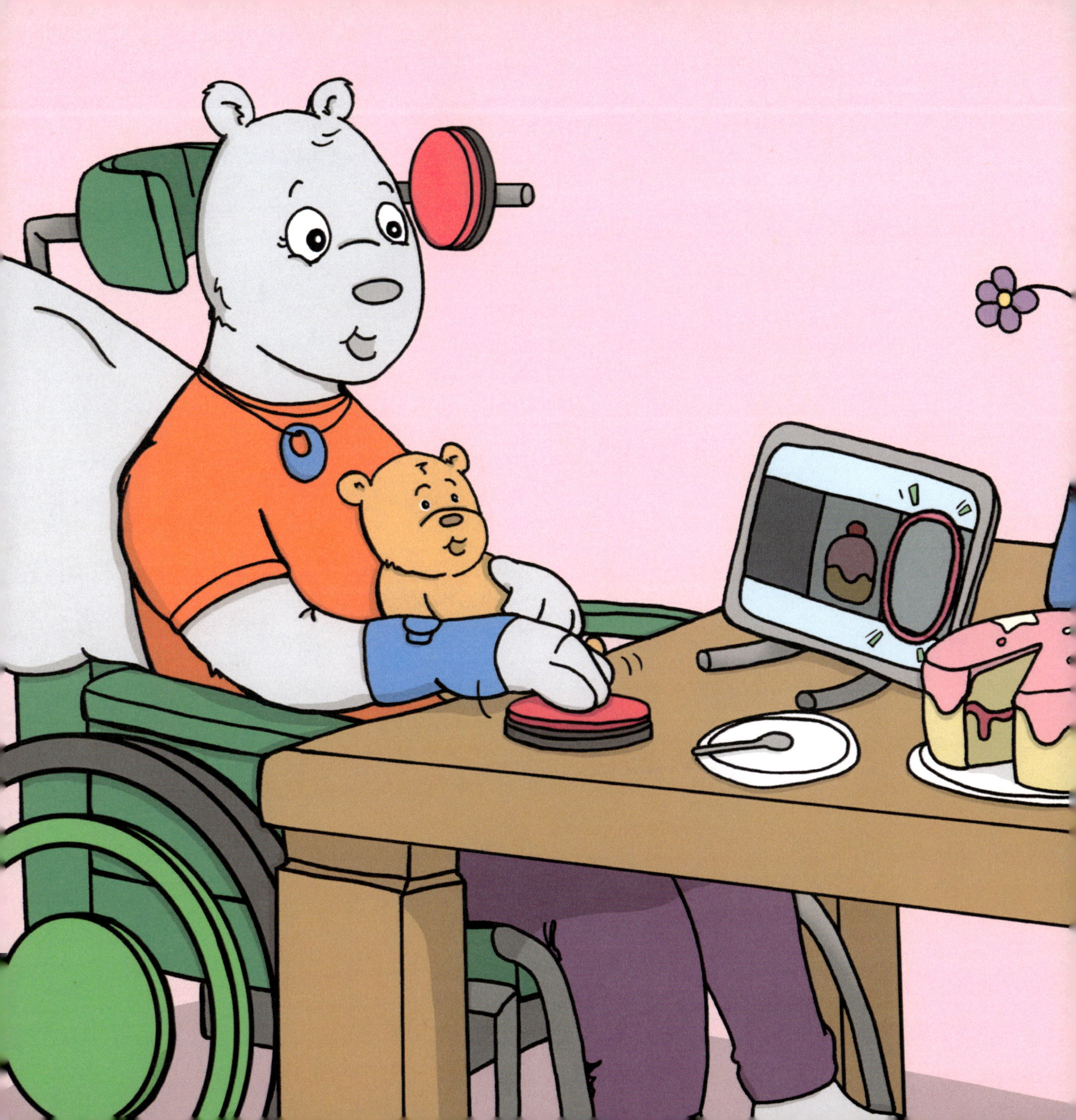

She confidently scans

And finds the word "cake"

Because it doesn't matter

That last time she
made a mistake

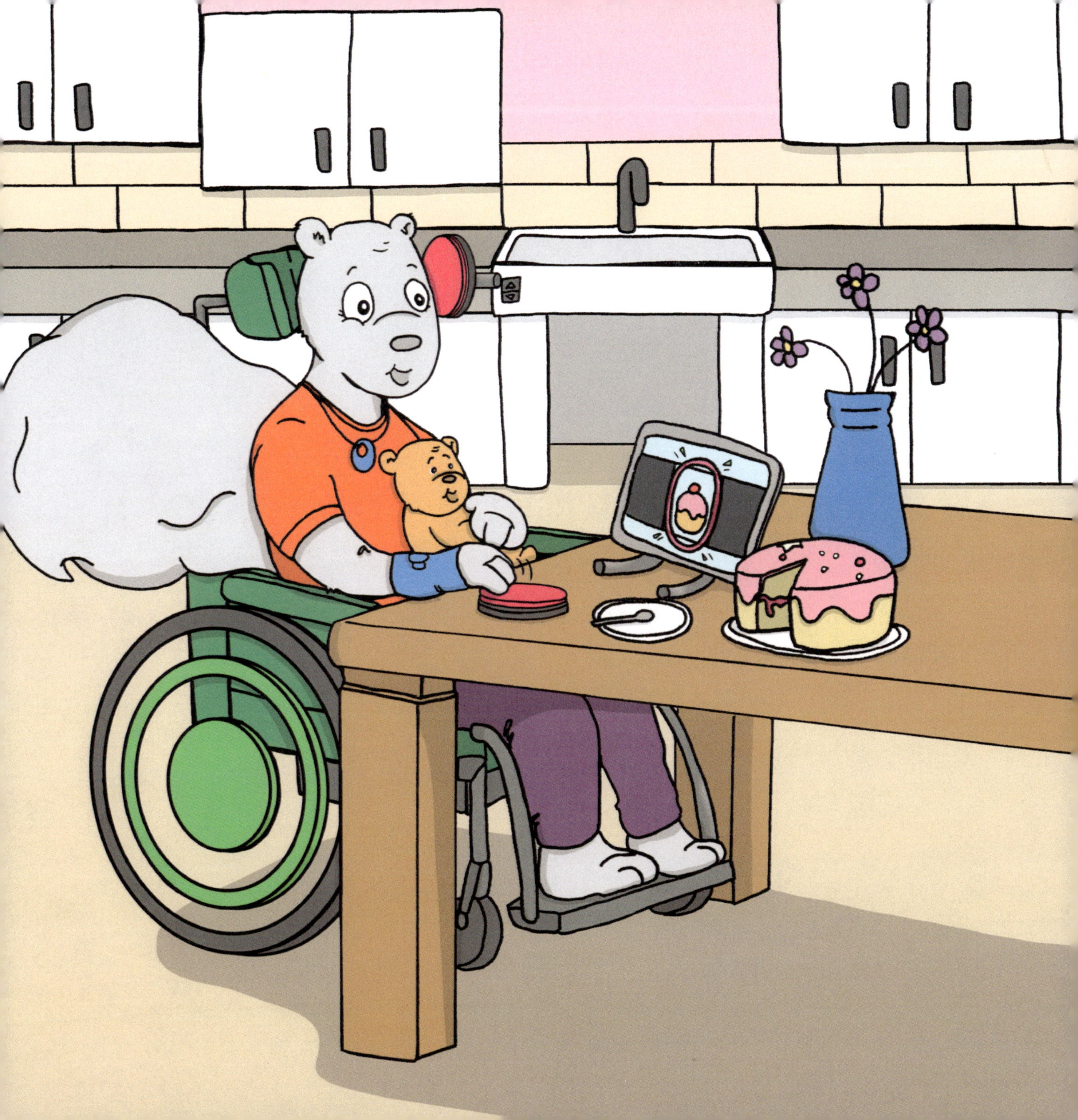

Now plug in your device

With increased vocabulary

Tell us how you're feeling

Connect with family!

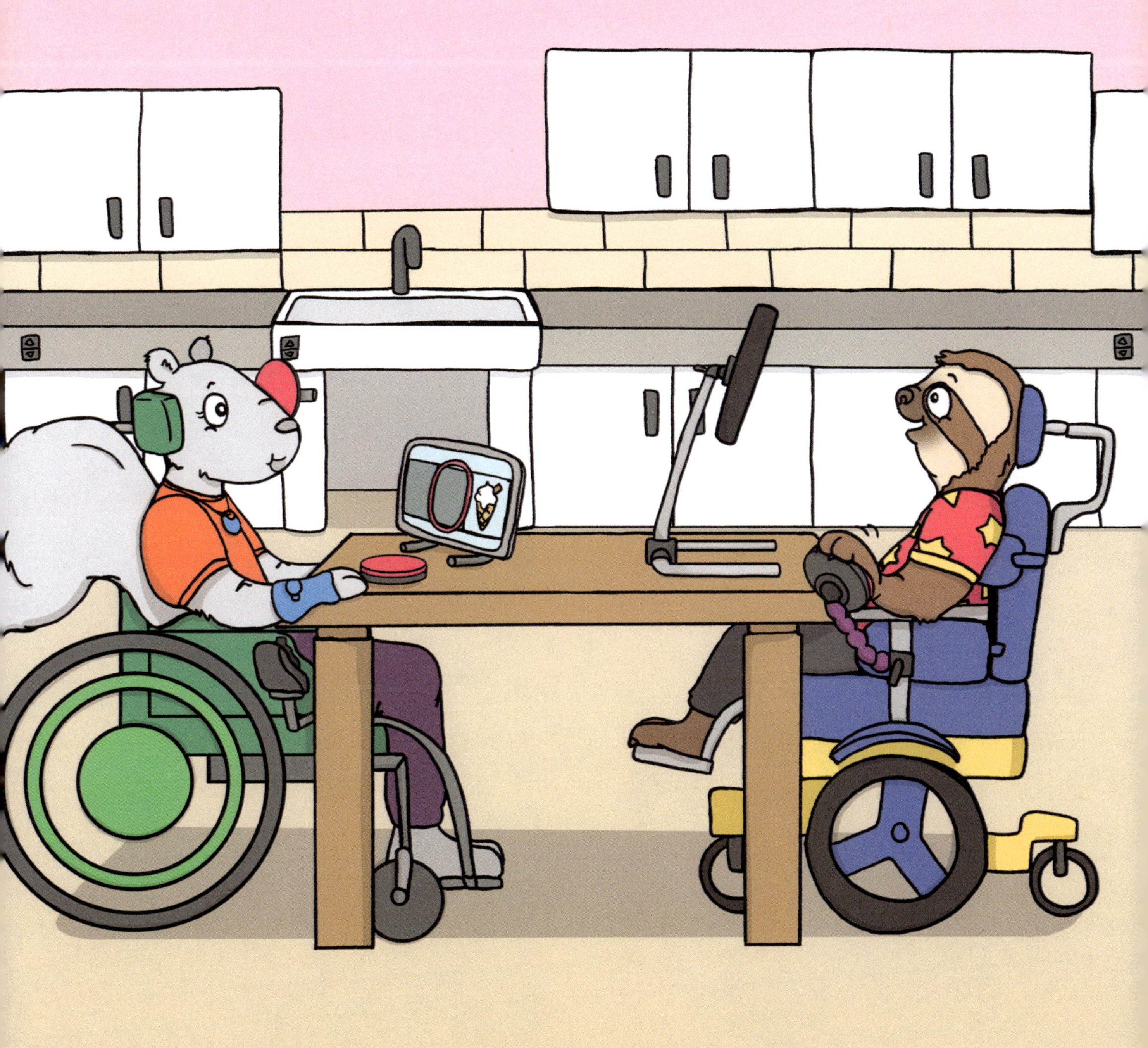

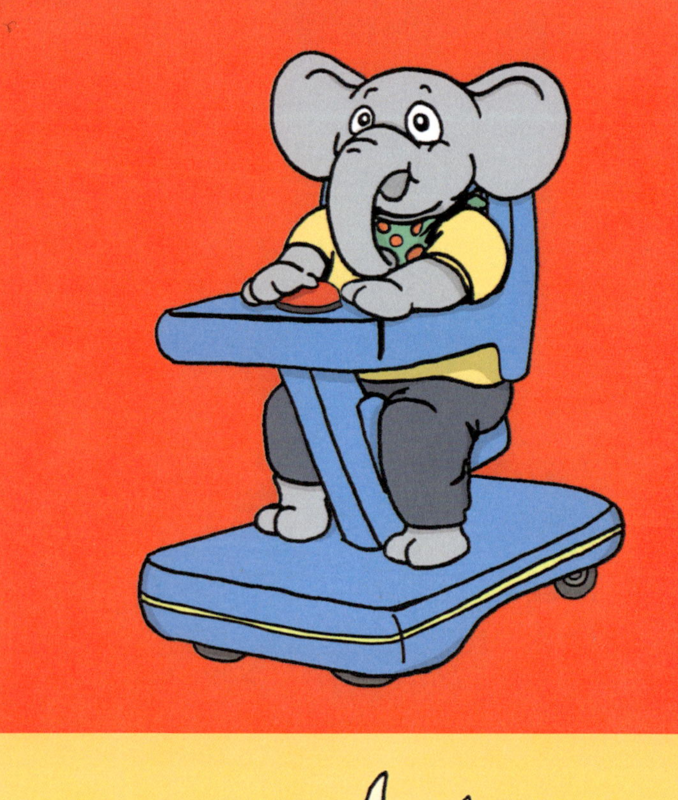
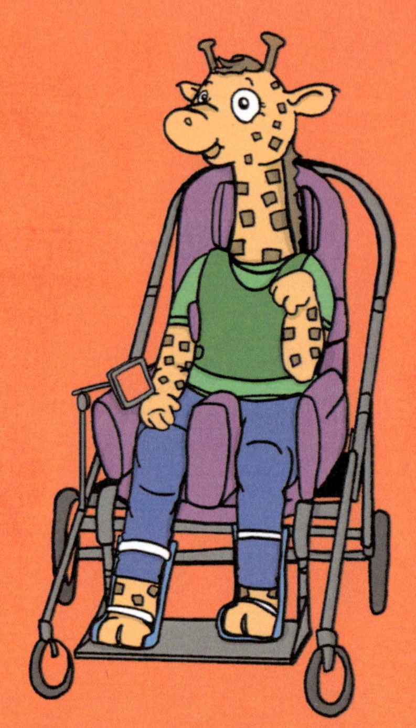
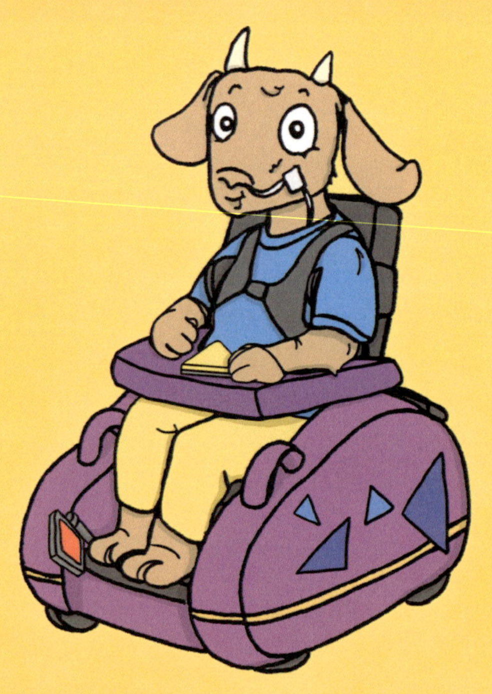
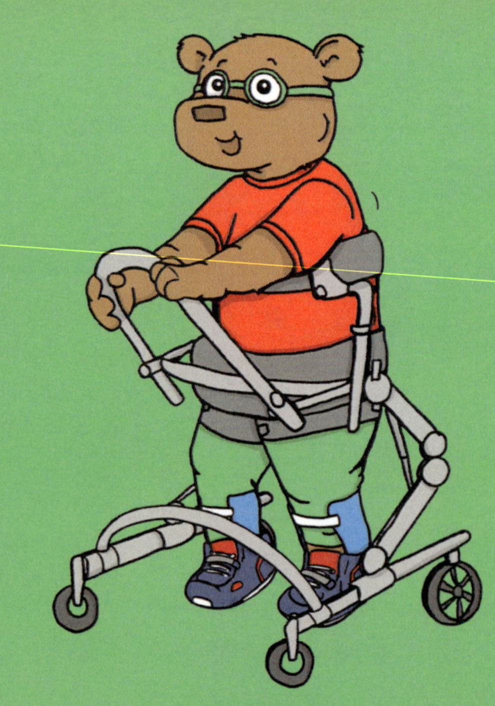

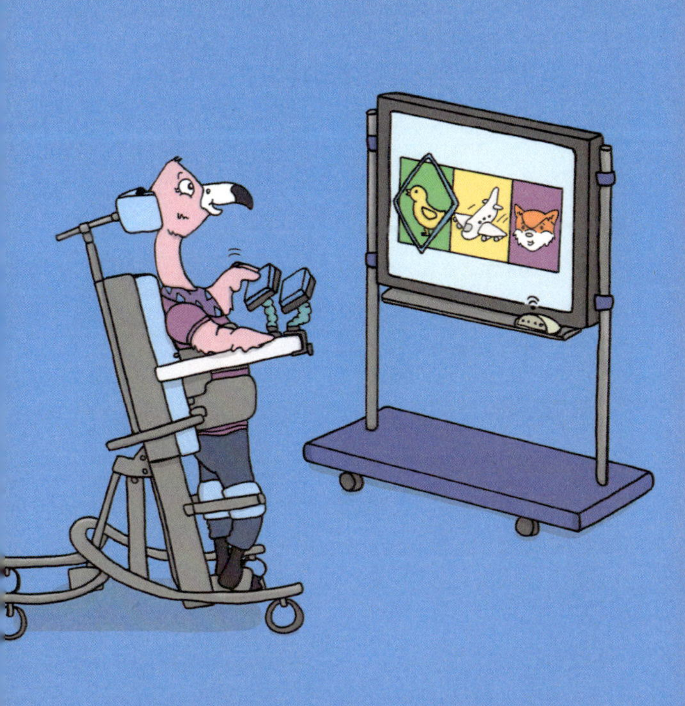

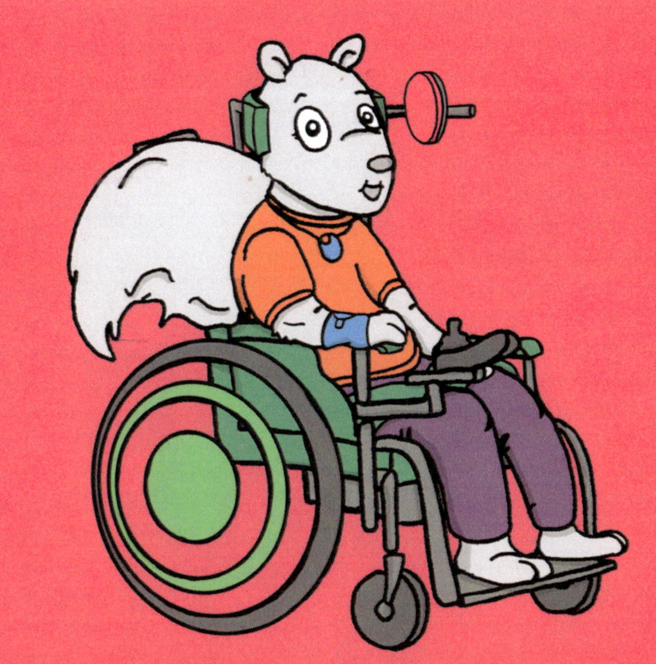

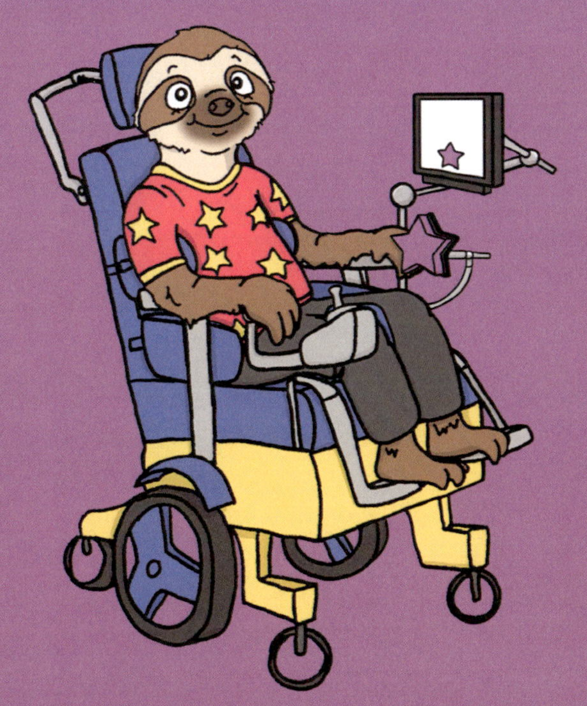

Photo of you!

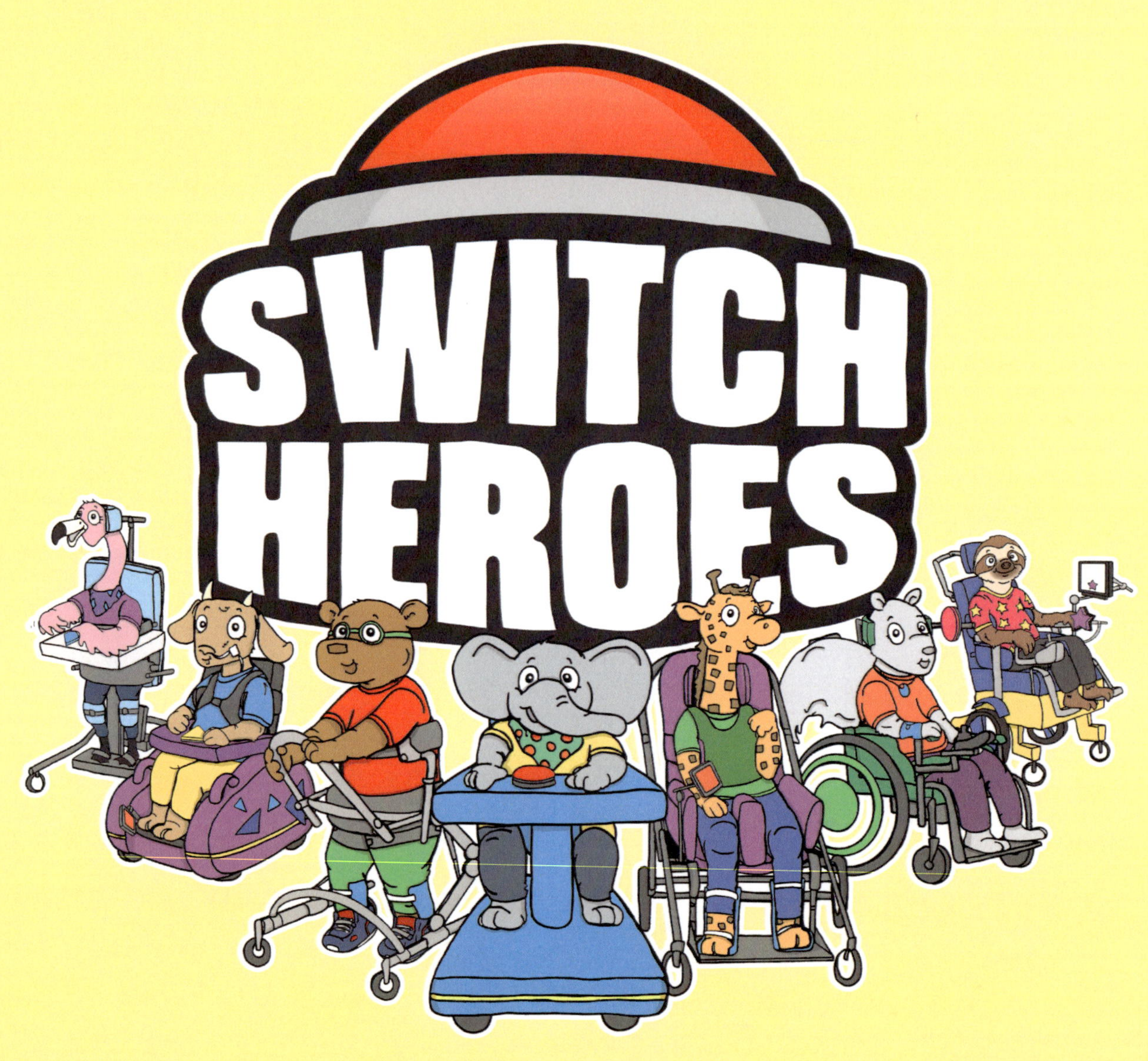

SWITCH
HEROES

The Seven Stages of Switch Development

The Seven Stages of Switch Development is a resource designed for switch-users, their families, caregivers and those who assist them in using switches. It features child-friendly characters and stories that support everyones learning.

The framework provides a helpful reference for measuring and tracking progress while offering flexibility to accommodate the unique needs and preferences of each switch-user.

Written directly to the switch-user, the framework can be read to them if they are unable to read it themselves. Our aim is to ensure that those supporting the child/switch-user can prioritise the child's needs and perspective in the process of developing their switch skills. We have seen the impact of involving the child in the learning process. Seeking their input and feedback regularly empowers them to take an active role in their development and combat learned helplessness.

Adapted from: Bean, I. (2011). Switch Progression Learning Journeys Road Map. Inclusive Technology. Burkhart, L. (2018). Stepping Stones to Switch Access. Perspectives of the ASHA Special Interest Groups, 3(12), pp.33-44. doi:https://doi/10.1044/persp3.sig12.33.

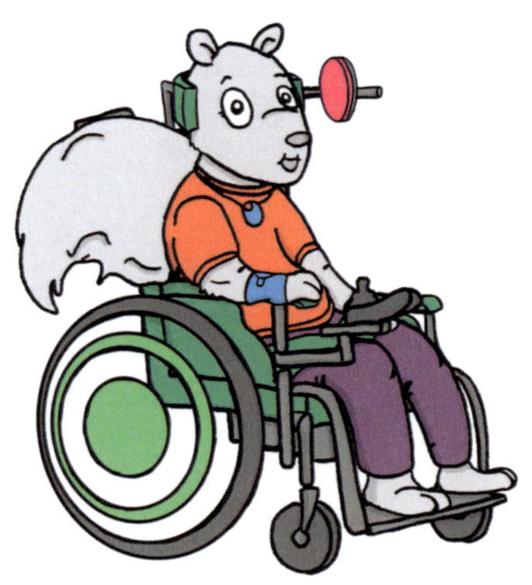

Stage 6
Using switch-scanning to find the right one
Succeeding Saffi the squirrel
Oval/Pink

Definition

Succeeding Saffi is the stage when you are ready to learn how to select the 'correct' option from a range of choices on the screen. To do this, you will need to use two switches to scan and select or one switch with timed input to make your choice. The aim of this stage is to help you learn how to make a specific choice instead of randomly selecting any option that is presented to you.

By taking your time and carefully considering the options before making a decision, you will become more discerning and intentional in your use of technology. This will help you to develop your decision-making skills and better understand the consequences of your choices.

Remember, the more you practise selecting the 'correct' option, the better you will become at using equipment and technology in general. So don't be afraid to try new things and keep learning!

Activity options can be graded based on the number of available choices (from few to many) and by leaving options blank or including incorrect options. For example, options can range from 'blank, blank, something' to 'incorrect, incorrect, correct.'

Milestones

- You have learnt to scan through options using two switches or just one with timed scanning

- You can identify and select the correct option from an increasing set of choices, differentiating between blank options, content options, and incorrect options

- You demonstrate your ability to use switch scanning for purposeful communication or participation in activities

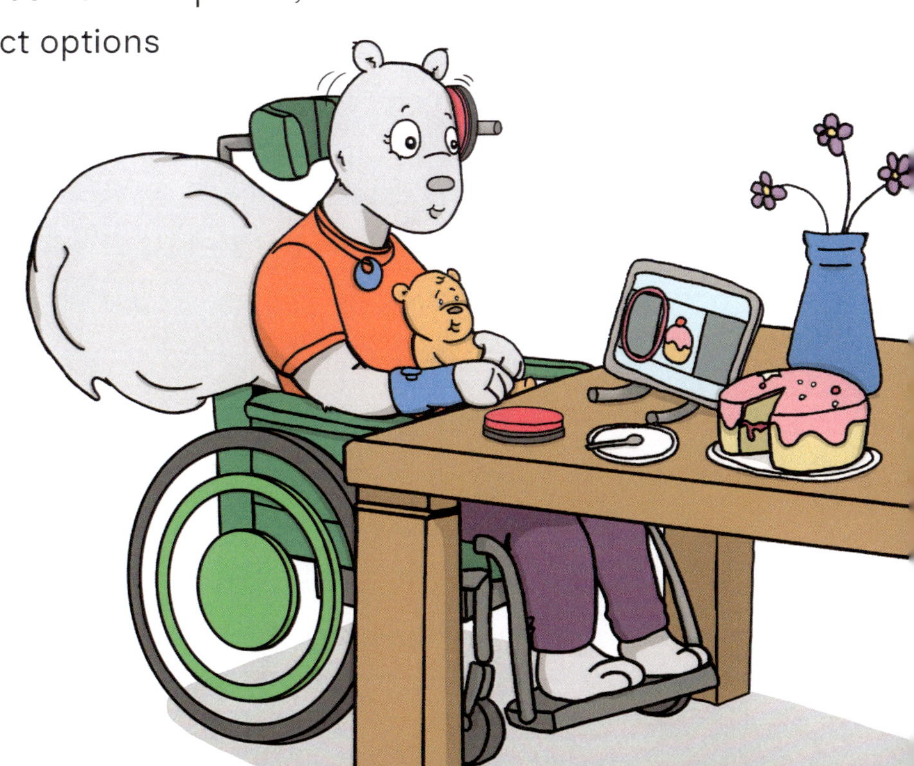

- Select an activity or item. Setup a grid on a communication device with three boxes. Have two empty and one with the activity or item. Setup multiple pages like this with different activities

- Use computer software with scanning choices on the screen for social interaction - directing an adult, sensory play, etc

- Communication apps: Use apps that incorporate scanning to enable the user to select and communicate specific messages or responses, such as communication boards or AAC devices

- Interactive stories: Interactive stories that use scanning to allow the user to make choices and follow different story paths, such as choose-your-own-adventure books

- Educational apps: Use apps that incorporate scanning to enable the user to select and complete various educational activities, such as spelling or maths games

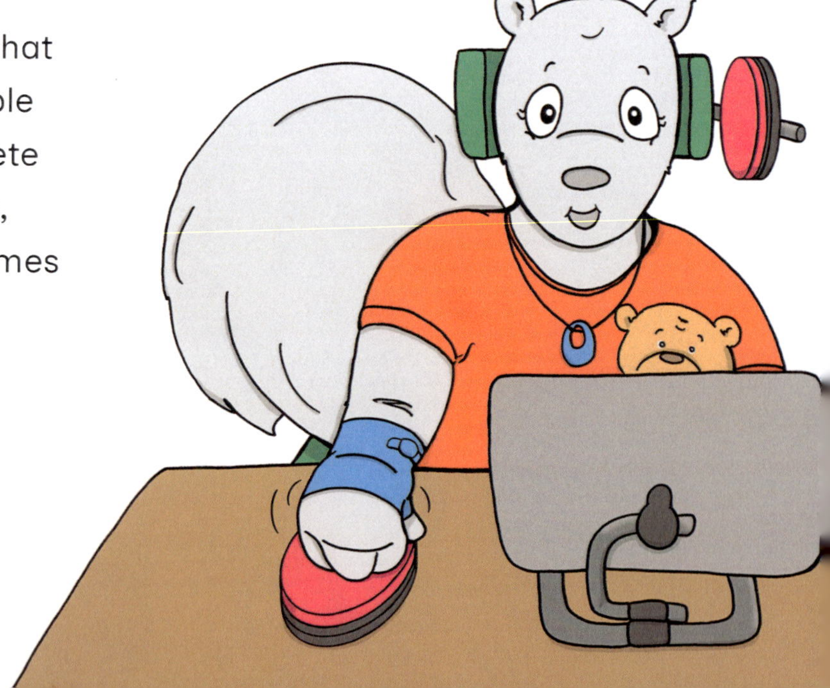

- Ask the child which option they would like to choose without using switches initially and then support them to find this option using their scanning and select switches

- Provide clear visual cues to help the user identify and select the correct option

- Encourage the user to practise visual discrimination by locating objects in their field of view with verbal prompting

- Use activities and materials that are motivating and engaging for the user

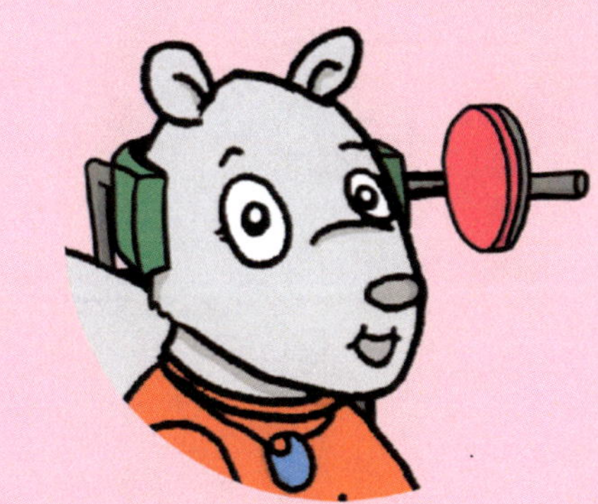

Instead of a prompt hierarchy where the type of prompt increase in support level, we recommend our one prompt switch support cycle. Find out more at Jiao.life

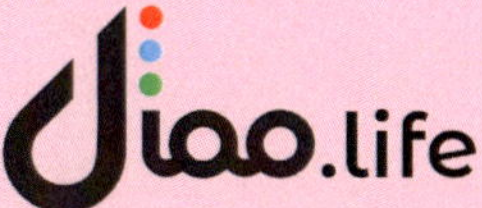

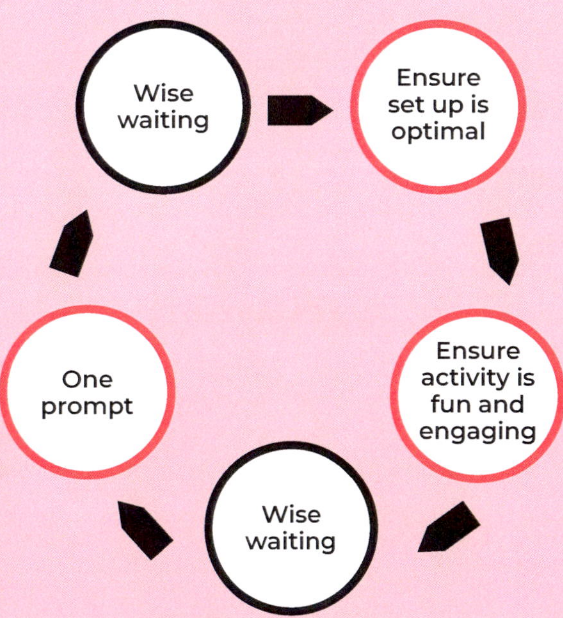

The Assessment Tool

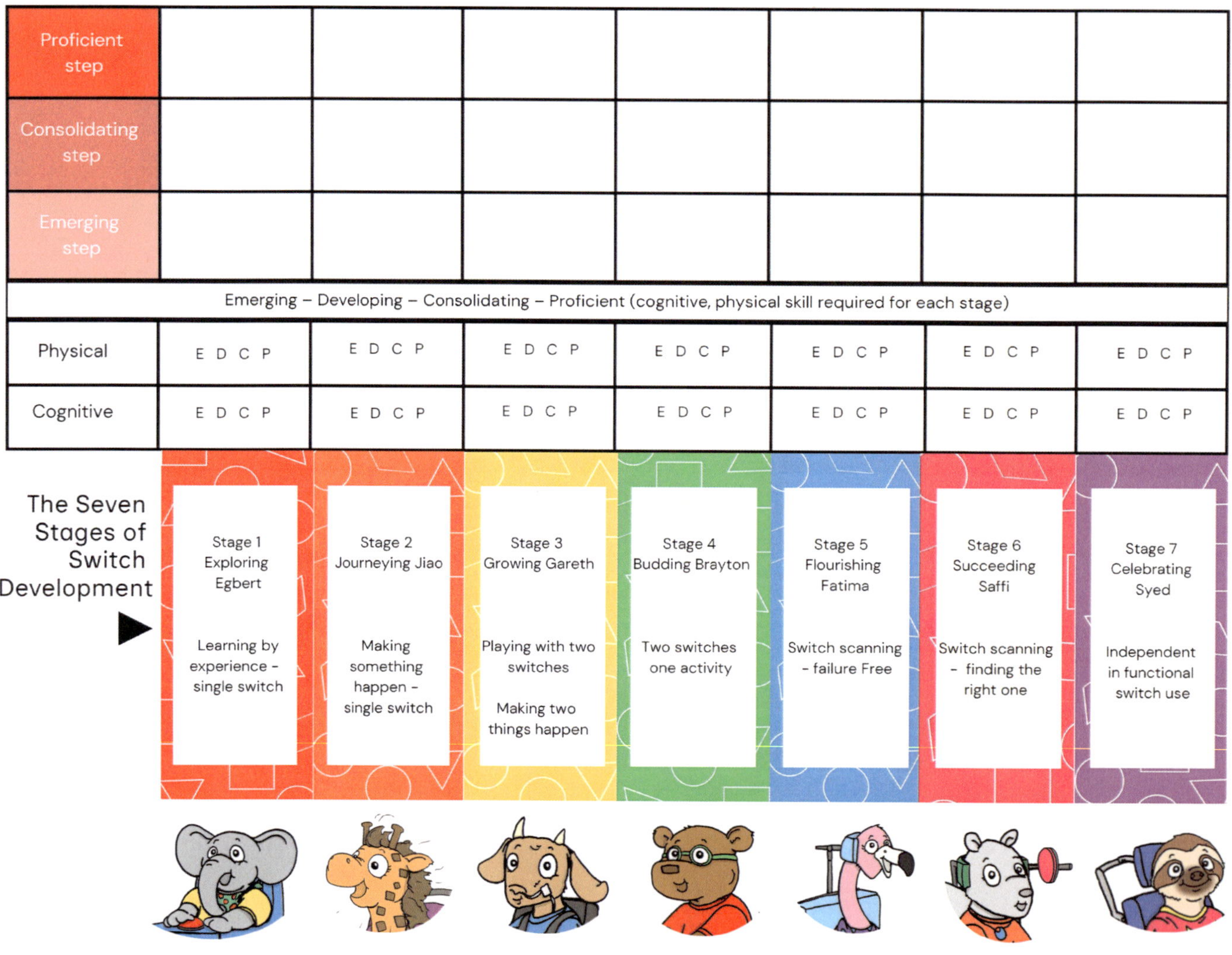

Print version available at Jiao.life

How to use the assessment tool

- The stages of switch development are not mutually exclusive, so progress can be made across multiple stages simultaneously

- Once a step is completed, mark it off and add the date

- The assessment tool can be used for goal setting, where helpers can add target dates and change the text/box colour accordingly

- There is a stream for assessing cognitive and physical skill development, divided into four steps for each stage (Emerging, Developing, Consolidating and Proficient)

- Helpers should consider the cognitive and physical skills required for each level

- This additional stream can help identify areas that may require additional support and highlight strengths and weaknesses for targeted interventions

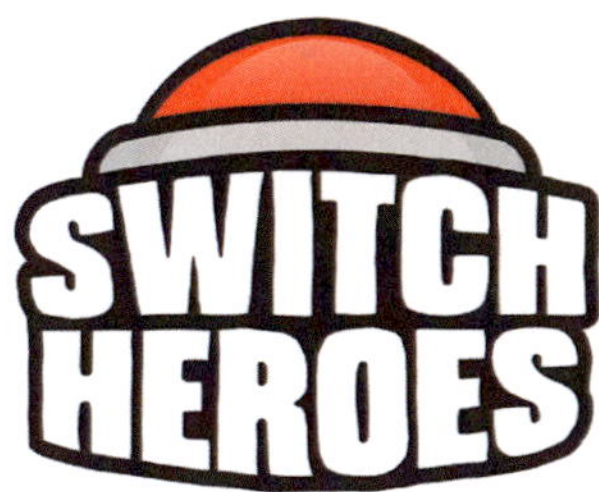

At Jiao Ltd, we are dedicated to empowering individuals through innovative assistive technology solutions.

We provide personalised services and training to help children, families, and professionals navigate the world of assistive tech. For more resources, training options, or to learn how we can support you, visit Jiao.life or get in touch with us directly. We look forward to hearing from you!

This is to certify that

____

is using switch scanning
to find the right one

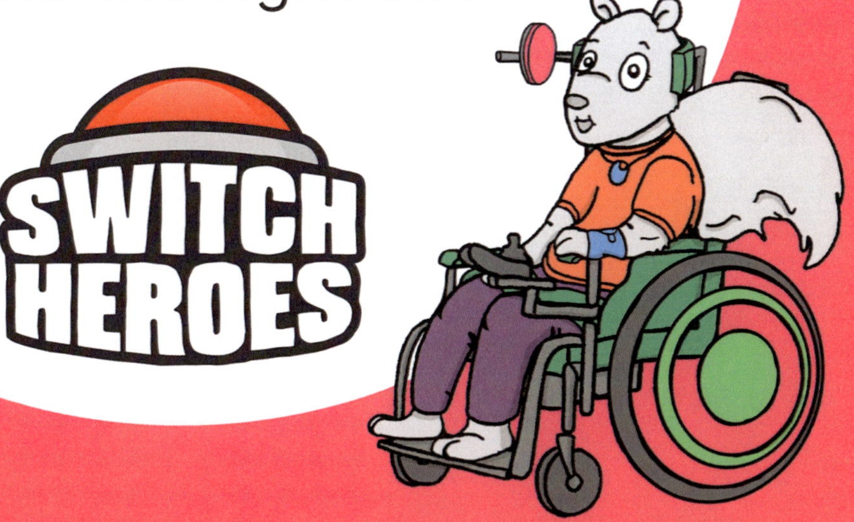

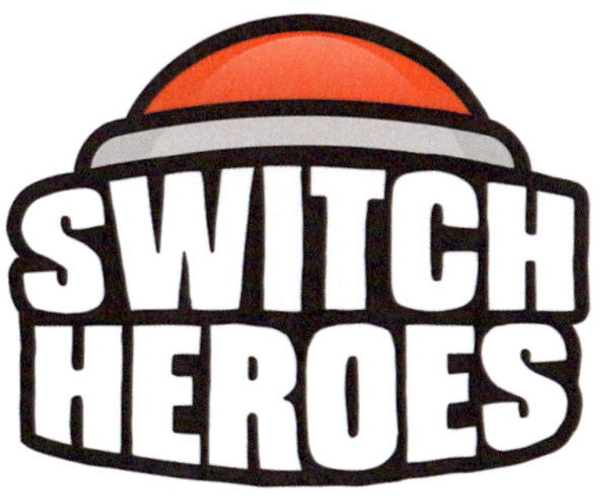